I0478426

CAREER AS A PHYSICAL THERAPIST

PHYSICAL THERAPY ASSISTANT

A YOUNG MOTHER STRUGGLES WITH MULTIPLE SCLEROSIS. A teenager sustains a concussion playing football. A soldier loses a leg. A child is born with cerebral palsy. An elderly man suffers a stroke. Thanks to the efforts of physical therapists, the young mother can now hold her child without fear of falling. The teenager is no longer experiencing dizziness and headaches. The soldier learns to walk normally with a prosthesis. The child takes her first step. The elderly man regains function and resumes daily activities.

Physical therapists, sometimes called PTs, play a major role in the diagnosis, treatment, and rehabilitation of people with all kinds of injuries, illnesses, and chronic conditions. The most common goal is to help people improve their movement and manage their pain. Treatment plans may include a combination of exercise, traction, mobilization, muscle manipulation, ultrasound, electrotherapy, vestibular training, motor development, and patient education. Assistive and adaptive devices may be used, such as crutches, wheelchairs, orthotics, and prosthetics. An important component of physical therapy is teaching an individual how to move or perform particular tasks in ways that will speed recovery and prevent further injury.

Physical therapy, which has been evolving for more than 200 years, can treat a wider range of problems with greater success than ever before. Today, there are many different kinds of physical therapy. Which kind is needed depends on the type of health problem. For example, a patient recovering from a heart attack needs different care than an athlete with a sports injury.

Physical therapists are trained to be able to treat all kinds of patients. Because there are so many different kinds, many PTs specialize in one particular area, such as orthopedics or pediatrics. A physical therapist can become board certified in any of nine areas, but there are many more specialties that can be practiced without certification.

Physical therapists must earn a Doctor of Physical Therapy (DPT) degree and become licensed to practice in their state. In total, it takes seven years of intense schooling after high school graduation to get to that point. Is it worth the time and hard work? Absolutely, say those in the field. In fact, physical therapy has been consistently ranked among the best careers to pursue. At a glance, the over 35 percent job growth over the next 10 years is exceptional. PTs are needed everywhere and the demand is far outpacing supply. Salaries are also good, generally ranging from $85,000 to $100,000 a year. The single reason most PTs are happy in their careers is the enormous satisfaction they get from helping people return to normal, fulfilling lives.

Are you looking for a career that offers great job security and the opportunity to earn a comfortable living? If you are compassionate, patient, and physically fit, read on. Physical therapy may be what you are looking for.

WHAT YOU CAN DO NOW

START BY VISITING THE AMERICAN Physical Therapy Association (APTA) website to find a list of accredited schools. Contact your top choices and ask for their admissions information. Then plan your high school curriculum carefully to make sure you meet all requirements. All college PT programs include numerous science courses. To prepare for that, take challenging courses in physics, biology, and chemistry in high school. Include as many AP

(Advanced Placement) courses as you can. Classes in social science, math, psychology, and any classes involving health are also good choices. Keep your grades above a 3.0 GPA.

A college physical therapy program is long and rigorous. Before making such a big commitment, make sure physical therapy is what you really want to do. You can begin to determine that by talking to professional physical therapists about their work. Ideally, you would job shadow several PTs in different settings. Your guidance counselor can help you make arrangements or you can simply call PTs in your town and ask to job shadow for a day or two. This is a good way to get a realistic understanding of what the work is like on a daily basis. Be observant and prepared to ask questions so you know what you will be getting into.

Get some hands-on experience. Look for volunteer work at a hospital, clinic, or other healthcare facility. You can also try to get a part-time job in a physical therapist's office. No special education or certification is needed to work as a physical therapist aide, but it does require a high school diploma. There are other roles you can fill even before you graduate. Approach the coaches at your school about working with one of the teams. You could supervise warm ups, record injuries, and track responses to treatments.

Start getting in shape. Physical therapists need strength and stamina. Getting involved in dance or any kind of sport will provide you with firsthand knowledge about the body's strengths, limits, and vulnerabilities. If possible, work with a personal trainer. In addition to getting fit, you will learn about body mechanics and sports injuries.

HISTORY OF THE CAREER

AS A PROFESSION, PHYSICAL THERAPY has been around for about 200 years in the US, but various forms of physiotherapy have been used in other countries since ancient times. Around 460 BC, Hippocrates prescribed manual therapy techniques such as massage to address stress and discomfort for patients in Greece. About the same time, Hector advocated the therapeutic use of water (hydrotherapy) to treat patients. There is also evidence that healers in ancient Egypt, China, and Persia advocated massage, exercise and movement for treatment of various physical ailments.

In 1813, Per Henrik Ling in Sweden founded the first professional group for physical therapists, the Royal Central Institute of Gymnastics. Ling's patient records tracked the results of patients who were treated with manipulative therapy techniques combined with exercise to overcome physical problems and injuries. At first, all patients were gymnasts. In fact, the Swedish word for physical therapist is *sjukgymnast,* which means "someone involved in gymnastics for those who are ill." There are documents showing that wealthy Americans traveled to Sweden for treatment that was not available in the US. In 1887, Sweden recognized physical therapy as an official profession. Other countries soon followed.

Four nurses in Great Britain formed the Chartered Society of Physiotherapy in 1894. The organization's purpose was to provide training in the known physical therapy techniques that existed at the time. Soon, other schools around the world followed the Society's example. Among them was the School of Physiotherapy at the University of Otago in New Zealand (1913) and Walter Reed Hospital in Washington DC, after the breakout of World War I (1914).

The evolution of physical therapy practice in the early 20th century was directly related to two global events: poliomyelitis epidemics and several major wars. Walter Reed Hospital graduated the first physical therapists during the First World War. These were nurses, then called Reconstruction Aides, who were trained to restore physical function to injured soldiers. Soon after, orthopedic surgeons began using physical therapy techniques to treat children with disabilities. These treatments were refined and applied during the polio outbreak of 1916. Both polio and physical injuries to war veterans would dominate the attention of physical therapists for the next 35 years.

Research became an important catalyst for the physical therapy movement in the 1920s. The first physical therapy research was published in the US in 1921 in the first edition of *The PT Review*. That same year, Mary McMillan established the Physical Therapy Association (now called the American Physical Therapy Association (APTA). It established educational standards for university professional PT programs. Now that training programs were being accredited by a national body, scientific research and technology would shape the profession. Members of the APTA got fully involved in medical research, including the Salk Vaccine Trials, which led to the end of polio epidemics in 1956.

Physical therapy treatment up through the 1940s mostly consisted of basic exercise, massage, and traction. The art of manipulative therapy had been abandoned for nearly 70 years. That changed and rapid progress ensued starting in the early 1950s. Manipulative procedures to the spine and extremity joints resurfaced, especially in the British Commonwealth countries.

In the US, the role of the physical therapist evolved from that of a technician to a professional healthcare practitioner. A growing number of states during the 1950s and 1960s enacted legislation that recognized physical therapy as a professional practice. Amendments to the Social Security Act (SSA) in 1967 added a definition of "outpatient physical therapy services."

Physical therapy started to move beyond hospitals. Although the majority of therapists continued to practice in hospitals through the 1960s, by the late 1950s many had started to practice in other settings, such as outpatient orthopedic clinics, public schools, colleges and universities, community health centers, geriatric settings (skilled nursing facilities), and rehabilitation centers.

In the 1960s and 1970s, physical therapy practices expanded to include more types of physical problems. The cardiopulmonary field benefitted from an increasing use of chest physical therapy treatment programs for patients, both before and after surgeries. The practice of physical therapy for patients with neuromuscular disorders also dramatically changed. With hip and other joint replacements becoming commonplace, new avenues for orthopedic physical therapy practice emerged. Certified specialization for physical therapists became available starting in 1974 with the Orthopedic Section of the APTA. In the same year, the International Federation of Orthopaedic Manipulative Therapy (IFOMT) was formed, which signaled coming change and progress in manual therapy worldwide. Physical therapists began providing services in the areas of women's health, oncology, and hand rehabilitation.

In the 1980s, the tidal wave of new technology led to major advances in rehabilitation with the introduction of computerized modalities such as ultrasound, electric stimulation, and iontophoresis.

In the 1990s, the Americans with Disabilities Act and the National Center for Medical Rehabilitation Research led to new opportunities for practice. Physical therapists were faced with the challenges of increasing governmental cost savings, decreasing reimbursement, increasing governmental regulations, and the influences of the insurance industry and corporate America.

In the new millennium, technical advances have continued to grow. One of the latest advances was in therapeutic cold laser, which gained FDA approval in the United States in 2002. The APTA developed a CD-ROM version and then the downloadable

PDF of the *Guide to Physical Therapist Practice*. The APTA's "Hooked-on-Evidence" project, initiated in 2002, was a groundbreaking step in APTA's mission to provide access to evidence-based information for PTs located anywhere in the world.

Today, physical therapists are continuing to find more ways to apply their skills, from aquatic treatment for elite athletes to children with developmental disabilities. As the field expands, so do the number of opportunities. The demand for services is far outpacing the number of qualified physical therapists and that demand will exist for the foreseeable future.

WHERE YOU WILL WORK

THERE ARE ABOUT 211,000 PHYSICAL THERAPISTS at work in the US. Most are employed by:

- Offices of physical, occupational and speech therapists, and audiologists
- Hospitals, public and private
- Home healthcare services
- Nursing and residential care facilities
- Offices of physicians

Historically, most physical therapists have worked in hospitals. There are three basic types of hospital-based care: acute care, rehabilitation, and extended care.

Acute care is provided in private and public hospitals to people who need short-term care due to illness, surgery, an accident, or recovery from a trauma. When patients need more time for rehabilitation, they are transferred to a long-term care facility, which may be either a rehabilitation hospital or a special hospital that provides medical and rehabilitation care specific to their needs.

Extended care is provided in skilled nursing facilities, nursing homes, and extended care facilities. Physical therapists in these settings typically care for elderly patients and people who are permanently disabled.

Although many physical therapists still work in hospitals, more than 80 percent now practice in other settings. These include the following:

Outpatient Clinics

This is the most common setting for a physical therapy practice today. Outpatient clinics are typically private practices that address less serious conditions that do not require hospitalization. Patients typically need help recovering from broken bones, severe sprains, pulled tendons, torn muscles, or other relatively minor injuries.

Sports and Fitness Facilities

Sports medicine has been growing in popularity for years. Physical therapists specializing in this type of work focus more on the prevention of injury rather than rehabilitation after an injury has occurred. People in their care are considered clients, not patients. Services are provided in fitness centers, public gyms, and all kinds of sports training facilities. Some PTs are hired by private sports consulting groups to work with professional athletes. In this case, they would be involved both in training and short-term rehabilitation.

Home Health

A growing number of physical therapists work for home health agencies. Home health PTs provide their services in the patient's home, caregiver's home, group home, residential facility, skilled nursing facility, or elsewhere in the community. The majority of patients are senior citizens. Other patients include children with developmental or physical disabilities, and individuals of all ages who have limited mobility or cannot fully function independently.

Corporate Employee Health Centers

In this setting, there is little hands-on therapy involved since the physical therapy services are focused on wellness and the prevention of illness and injury in the workplace. Physical therapists do this by promoting a healthy lifestyle with an emphasis on proper nutrition and exercise. They also teach individuals how to improve safety and recognize their physical limits.

Hospice

In the hospice setting, physical therapists help patients who are in the final days of life. The focus is on quality of life, however long or short that may be. The physical therapist helps patients to manage their pain and discomfort while maintaining functional abilities for as long as possible.

Government Health Agencies

Physical therapists work for all levels of government, from local to federal. Depending on the employing agency, services may be provided to civilians or military personnel. The largest agencies hiring physical therapists at the federal level include the Veteran's Health Administration (VHA), Department of Defense, and Indian Health Service (IHS).

Private Research Facilities

Research centers hire physical therapists to collaborate with other professionals to find new ways to improve patient care outcomes and support the body of knowledge in the field of physical therapy. Research facilities are usually (but not always) associated with pharmaceutical and medical device manufacturers.

Physical therapists can also be found working for community

health centers, organizations for the handicapped, and schools of all kinds.

About 20 percent of physical therapists are self-employed. They may work from home and use part of their own residence as their office space, but not for treatment. They may choose from a variety of facilities, such as local gyms or group practice offices, as a place to meet and treat their clients.

Most physical therapists work full time on a regular Monday-to-Friday schedule. In some settings, such as hospitals, it may be necessary to work evening or weekend shifts. About one out of five PTs work part time.

THE WORK YOU WILL DO

PHYSICAL THERAPISTS DIAGNOSE AND TREAT PEOPLE who have functional problems resulting from birth defects, back and neck injuries, sprains and strains, fractures, chronic diseases like arthritis or asthma, amputations, neurological disorders such as stroke or cerebral palsy, work and sports related injuries, and more. Patients include individuals of all ages, from newborns to the very oldest, who are in pain or have difficulty moving and performing everyday activities. PTs also work with individuals to prevent the loss of mobility before it occurs by developing fitness and wellness programs that promote healthier and more active lifestyles.

Physical therapists are capable of treating a broad variety of people and conditions, but the same basic five-step procedure is applied to every patient.

Step 1: Examination and Assessment

Many patients come with a diagnosis from their referring physician, but the PT does not rely on that. The initial visit starts with a review of the patient's medical history, including medications, test results, and any notes from other healthcare providers. Then the PT conducts a thorough examination, performing tests to measure muscle function, strength, joint flexibility, range of motion, balance and coordination, posture, respiration, skin integrity, motor function, quality of life, and the ability to perform normal activities of daily living.

Step 2: Diagnosis

The PT identifies issues that need attention based on test results, through observation, and by listening to the patient's concerns. A complete diagnosis covers the patient's current status as well as a projected goal for treatment. The physical therapist will also determine when and how the patient will be able to reintegrate into the workforce or community.

Step 3: Plan

Once a diagnosis has been determined, the physical therapist designs a plan of care. Every plan is customized for the individual patient, taking into account their specific goals and unique situation. Plans are based on the PT's medical expertise and experience along with the best available research. Both short and long-term projections are outlined. The PT will determine which therapeutic modalities and interventions, such as assistive or adaptive devices, will be utilized. At this point, the PT will explain the plan and teach the patient the best ways to prevent further injury or complications until treatment is complete. Once the patient thoroughly understands what to do and what to expect, treatment will begin.

Step 4: Treatment

Therapeutic exercise and functional training form the foundation of every physical therapist treatment, but they are rarely the only components. For example, hands-on therapy may be used to manipulate joints or massage muscles to promote proper movement and function. Other external stimulation techniques include application of heat or cold, hydrotherapy, traction, ultrasound, infrared or ultraviolet light, and electrical stimulation. The physical therapist might also prescribe the use of assistive devices, such as canes, crutches, prosthetics, wheelchairs, and walkers to help with mobility. These devices are also used during therapeutic exercise routines. For example, a patient with a spinal injury might walk on a treadmill while being supported by a harness.

Step 5: Monitoring

Throughout the course of treatment, the PT carefully tracks the patient's progress. The patient is re-examined periodically to determine if treatments are working as planned. If not, the plan may be modified to include new, more effective treatments. It may take weeks, months, or even years to achieve the desired outcome. Throughout the process, the PT educates patients and their families about what to expect and how to cope with the challenges that will inevitably occur.

Specialties

Physical therapists are highly trained to treat a wide range of physical conditions. Some choose to practice as generalists, applying their skills to all kinds of situations. Many others prefer to specialize in particular areas of clinical practice. There are many different types of physical therapy to choose from, but currently there are certifications for nine.

Cardiovascular & pulmonary rehabilitation therapists treat patients with problems affecting the heart or lungs. Some treatments are long term, such as using manual therapy to help clear lung secretions caused by cystic fibrosis. More often, the goal is to rebuild endurance and functional independence in patients who have experienced heart attacks or have undergone cardiac surgery, such as a coronary bypass.

Clinical electrophysiology is a specialty area that focuses on electrotherapy and wound management. It is a growing area because physical therapy techniques have been proven to greatly increase the quality of life for patients with chronic, non-healing wounds. Electrotherapy in particular can maximize overall function and range of motion in cases of compromised skin integrity.

Geriatrics physical therapy covers a wide range of issues experienced by older adults. Some common examples include arthritis, osteoporosis, cancer, Alzheimer's disease, hip and joint replacement, balance disorders, and incontinence.

Neurological physical therapy is concerned with the broad array of neurological disorders, such as stroke, chronic back pain, cerebral palsy, multiple sclerosis, Parkinson's disease, and spinal cord injuries. PT specialists help patients with these and other conditions overcome impairments of vision, balance, ambulation, movement, muscle strength, and functional independence.

Oncology physical therapy plays a critical role during all stages of cancer care. Surviving cancer requires a motivating, encouraging, and positive environment. PTs provide that and much more. Therapy is focused on optimizing function and quality of life. For example, they help patients proactively manage side effects of treatments, maintain strength, overcome fatigue, minimize pain, and generally maximize functional abilities. Oncology PTs also apply gentle but effective treatment for end-of-life care.

Orthopedic physical therapists deal with disorders and injuries of the musculoskeletal system (muscles, bones, ligaments, and tendons). Treatments, which are usually provided in an outpatient clinic, typically address fractures, acute sports injuries, arthritis, sprains, strains, back and neck pain, spinal conditions, tendinopathy, bursitis, amputations, and rehabilitation after orthopedic surgery. Techniques include joint manipulation, dry needling, muscle reeducation, hot/cold therapy, therapeutic exercise, and several types of electrical muscle stimulation.

Pediatric physical therapists treat infants, children, and adolescents for a variety of congenital, developmental, neuro-muscular, skeletal, or acquired diseases. They are particularly focused on early detection of health problems. Once a diagnosis is made, they use a selection of techniques designed to improve gross and fine motor skills, balance and coordination, strength and endurance, cognitive abilities, and sensory processing.

Sports therapy is a popular area for physical therapists. These specialists provide care for athletes at all levels, both professional and recreational. Treatment usually involves injury management, including assessment and diagnosis of initial injury, application of treatment, progressive rehabilitation for full return to sport, and prevention education.

Women's health physical therapists are concerned with the female reproductive system. This may include prenatal, childbirth, and postpartum. Commonly treated conditions include pelvic pain, lymphedema, osteoporosis, and urinary incontinence. Manual therapy techniques have also been successfully used to increase rates of conception in women with infertility.

Physical Therapy Assistants and Aides

Physical therapists are helped by two kinds of workers: physical therapy aides and physical therapy assistants.

PT aides work under the direct supervision of a physical therapist or physical therapist assistant. This is an entry-level position that does not require certification, and training is provided on the job. The types of tasks that PT aides are allowed to perform vary by state, but typically they do the following:

- Clean and organize treatment areas

- Set up therapy equipment and prepare for each patient's session

- Wash linens and order supplies

- Help patients move to and/or from the therapy area

- Perform clerical tasks, such as answer phones, fill out insurance forms, and schedule treatments

Physical therapist assistants are also under the direction and supervision of physical therapists, but they are more involved in the direct care of patients. Their responsibilities commonly include:

Observe patients before, during, and after therapy

Record patient progress and report the results of each treatment to the physical therapist

Help patients do specific exercises prescribed by the PT

Apply a variety of therapeutic techniques, such as massage, stretching, gait, and balance training

Teach and help patients use devices and equipment, such as walkers

Educate patient and family members about what to do after treatment

PHYSICAL THERAPISTS TELL THEIR OWN STORIES

I Am a Traveling Physical Therapist

"Shortly before I graduated, my professor warned me that there was still a lot to learn about physical therapy. I was advised to look into traveling PT because it offered greater opportunities to learn additional skills than any traditional job ever could. After contacting a number of agencies, I learned it was particularly advantageous for new graduates. It helps new therapists ease the transition from school to full-time work.

I signed up with a smaller agency that only handles clients in my state. My first assignment put me in a clinic with an experienced therapist who acted as my temporary mentor. He helped me get started in real-world PT and gave me lots of encouragement. It was a lot like interning, with one big exception – the pay was excellent. First off, it pays real hourly wages, so rather being paid a set salary for 40 hours when it turns out to be 50 hours of work, every extra hour is paid for. The combination of a high hourly pay and housing and living allowances meant I could live comfortably while making a big dent in my student loans. I later learned that larger staffing firms offer more benefits, such as health insurance, that small companies can't match.

I have been traveling for two years now. In that time, I have been exposed to a wide variety of treatment styles and techniques and have built great professional relationships. I have been able to live and vacation in wonderful places, taking breaks whenever I wanted. Traveling PT has also given me the chance to see many different PT operating systems and management styles. That will be useful when and if I decide to settle down and commit to a single employer."

I Am a Pediatric Physical Therapist

"Being a pediatric physical therapist means I encourage children to move, to grow, and to become independent. I do that by dancing, singing, and jumping with my young clients. Yes, it's hard work, but I make sure the exercises and the whole therapy process is fun. Pediatric PT is as much about creativity as it is about clinical skills.

I treat infants, children and adolescents with a variety of injuries and health issues. It takes particular knowledge of human movement and development to recognize the beginning of mobility and health problems in children. Even after nearly 10 years of practice, I am still learning. Pediatrics is a specialty that requires me to stay up to date on the latest research.

PT work is satisfying, but working with children is especially rewarding. Every step forward feels like it deserves a standing ovation. None of it comes easily so I make sure no small victory goes unnoticed. There are days, though, that seem filled with crying babies, moody teenagers, and frustrated parents. Then there are other days when I am overloaded with paperwork. Finally, I see the excited face of a child taking a first step, and it fills me with pride."

I Am a Physical Therapy Assistant

"I work in a hospital with people who have been injured badly enough to warrant being admitted for a stay. The injuries are usually to the knee, hip, or head. Sometimes there are inner ear injuries that cause balance problems. I also see patients with Parkinson's, Alzheimer's, and Lou Gehrig's disease. I like the variety of working in a hospital. Some days are more challenging than others, but the work is always interesting and there isn't a lot of stress.

As a PT assistant, I'm not allowed to do any therapy work on my own. The law requires me to act under the direction of a physical therapist. In addition to assisting with treatments, I oversee PT aides who mostly do paperwork.

I became a PTA because I wanted satisfying work that paid reasonably well. Hospitals usually pay less than private practice clinics, but there is greater job security. I know I'll always have a job. I do earn a good living, especially considering it only took two years of school to get started. I get a great deal of satisfaction out of my work. I love being able to help people get back to their lives."

PERSONAL QUALIFICATIONS

ALL PHYSICAL THERAPISTS GRADUATE FROM COLLEGE with a wide range of skills and techniques that they have learned to use with patients. Did you ever wonder what sets successful PTs apart from the rest? Even the best student, with a head for math and science, needs an array of personality and character traits to do the job well. Take a look at these traits of successful PT pros. Do these traits describe you?

People Skills

Are you a people person? Do friends and relatives feel they can talk to you about their personal matters? Physical therapy is a profession that is centered on people – all types and ages of people. Effective PTs are comfortable around people, and have a natural flair for listening with a genuine concern for others. They work closely with patients and are able to help them feel at ease during therapeutic sessions. PTs also routinely deal with people other than patients, such as family members, caretakers, and other healthcare providers. Successful PTs work in a spirit of cooperation in order to ensure that the recovery process runs smoothly and efficiently.

Compassion

Physical therapists are drawn to the profession by a true desire to help people. The best PTs have a nurturing nature and deep empathy for their patients who are in pain. Patients often feel vulnerable, embarrassed, or depressed about their situation. There will be many personal, heart-to-heart moments that may be emotionally difficult for the therapist as well as the patient. Good PTs have a knack for showing concern and understanding while maintaining control of difficult sessions with strength and a sense of humor.

Strength

This is physically demanding work that requires stamina and a high-energy level. Throughout the day, PTs stoop, kneel, crouch, and stand for long periods of time. They use their hands to manipulate and massage muscles and joints. During sessions, patients have to be lifted, turned, and have their weight supported while doing rehabilitative exercises. Often, it is the physical therapist who is doing most of the work. Successful PTs are naturally inclined to live a healthy lifestyle themselves and exercise regularly to maintain their own fitness.

Positive Attitude

Physical therapy is hard work. Patients naturally get discouraged or even angry when struggling with difficult exercises that may make them worse before they feel better. Good PTs understand that physical therapy is as much mental as it is physical. They are optimists who naturally focus on what is working and improving, rather than what is not. They know that patients respond best to encouragement and someone who believes in them.

Patience

The recovery process can take a long time and sometimes the treatment is painful or difficult. Even short-term treatments can be tedious and discouraging. Some patients will want to give up, while others take out their frustrations on the therapist. In order to successfully complete therapy, they need a PT who has more patience than they do. The best PTs are able to remain steady and calm while continually offering encouragement and reassurance.

ATTRACTIVE FEATURES

YEAR AFTER YEAR, PHYSICAL THERAPY is ranked high among the best careers to pursue. Three out of four professionals in the field say they are very happy – even enthusiastic – about what they do for a living. What is so great about this career? Good pay, flexibility, and job satisfaction top the list, but there are other rewards as well. Take a look at what makes this career so attractive.

Making a Difference

Imagine being able to help someone return to a normal, fulfilling life after being badly injured in a car crash. The satisfaction is immeasurable. Every day, physical therapists work one-on-one with patients who are living miserable lives because of strokes, chronic disease, birth defects, or other catastrophic events. Over time, their treatments ease pain, restore mobility, and prevent long-term disability. Through the course of a career, a physical therapist touches the lives of many people, making a significant difference in each and every case.

Flexibility

Very few career paths are as flexible as physical therapy. You can choose to work in a variety of different settings, from local gyms to trauma centers to patients' homes. There are also a number of specialized areas to choose from like pediatrics, sports medicine, orthopedics, or oncology. Very few careers, especially in healthcare, allow workers to choose part-time or per diem schedules. Physical therapists can opt for flexible scheduling that allows for interests outside of work. There is also the option to be your own boss. More than one out of every five physical therapists are self-employed.

Go Anywhere

Physical therapy jobs are available all over the country, in cities, small towns, and rural locations. Choose where you want to live and chances are good you will find a job there. Are you ambitious? There are programs that offer general compensation packages to attract PTs to locations you might not have considered, such as Alaska. Want to travel the world? There are also programs that help physical therapists gain licensure in other countries. Feeling adventurous? Per diem PTs can travel just about anywhere, work as little or as much as they want, and get a pay bump in the process.

Job Security

Physical therapists are always needed, in good economic times and bad. The demand has been growing steadily and now the forecast is for a tremendous increase of over 35 percent in the number of job openings over the next 10 years. That means the field is expanding at a much faster rate than most other occupations. Opportunities are abundant now and physical therapists can feel secure in the knowledge there will always be people who need their help.

Reasonable Hours

Healthcare careers are notorious for demanding long hours at all times of the day and night. Doctors, nurses, and even physician assistants work grueling hours that often interfere with family time and special occasions, and not so for physical therapists. They rarely have to work outside the hours of 7am and 8pm. Those who do happen to work weekends or holidays typically come out way ahead with big pay bonuses and the chance to take time off during the week in exchange.

UNATTRACTIVE ASPECTS

THE WORK IS CERTAINLY REWARDING, but it is not for everyone. Not everyone has what it takes to complete the necessary education. Some people are not born with an aptitude for math and science. Others are uncomfortable with human anatomy subjects and learning to handle bodily functions. Then there are those who are not prepared to handle the years of clinical and laboratory studies required to become a physical therapist. Make no mistake, the training is tough. Only hard-working, dedicated students make it to graduation.

Physical therapy is physically demanding work. Not everyone is up to the challenge. PTs often have to use their own bodies to lift patients who cannot move, which makes them vulnerable to back injuries. They also need strong hands to manually manipulate muscles and tendons that resist movement. They spend most of their time on their feet, which is tiring by itself. Successful PTs maintain a healthy diet, get ample sleep, and learn to use proper body mechanics and lifting techniques to avoid injuring themselves.

Physical therapists also need to be emotionally fit. Most patients in need of physical therapy have been through traumatic illnesses or injuries. Many have been in pain for long periods of time. Day after day, your job is to motivate them to do exercises that hurt and remind them of their limitations. Some will take their frustrations out on you and be unpleasant to work with. Others may refuse to follow the treatment plan designed to help them recover as quickly as possible. The emotional strain of working with people who are frustrated with their limited abilities can take its toll. It can be emotionally stressful and exhausting. PTs who are not emotionally strong enough to deal with witnessing the pain and suffering of patients every day may experience burnout.

Because of the huge demand for physical therapy services, opportunities are plentiful for newly licensed physical therapists. The job security is great, but there are few real advancement opportunities. The work you do will be about the same after 10 years in the field as it was in your first job out of college. Ambitious people who enjoy the challenge of climbing a career ladder to higher positions may have to settle for larger salaries. For those who enjoy the work, pay raises and stability are enough to keep them happy.

The paperwork can be tedious. About 10 percent of your time will be spent filling out insurance claim forms and filing progress reports

.

EDUCATION AND TRAINING

TO PRACTICE AS A PHYSICAL THERAPIST in the United States, you must earn a degree from an education program accredited by the Commission on Accreditation in Physical Therapy Education (CAPTE). There are currently more than 200 such programs, all of which offer only a Doctor of Physical Therapy (DPT) degree to new students. Most DPT programs require applicants to apply through the Physical Therapist Centralized Application Service (PTCAS).

Most programs require applicants to have a bachelor's degree prior to admission into the DPT program. There are usually specified educational prerequisites, such as classes in biology, chemistry, anatomy, physiology, and physics. Most DPT programs last three years. About 80 percent of the curriculum is classroom and lab study. The remaining 20 percent is hands-on clinical education. PT students complete at least 30 weeks of supervised clinical work, in areas such as acute care and orthopedic care. Coursework varies among the many DPT programs, but most include classes in biomechanics, behavioral sciences, kinesiology, exercise physiology, cellular histology, neuroscience, pharmacology, and evidence-based practice.

There are some six or seven year programs that allow students to graduate with both a bachelor's degree and a DPT. These typically work in a 3+3 format. The first three years consists of specific pre-professional (undergraduate/pre-PT) courses. Upon completion, students can advance into the second three-year professional DPT program. These combination programs allow high school graduates to apply. If accepted, students start as college freshmen and automatically advance into the professional phase of the PT program after completing specific undergraduate courses and complying with other stipulations, such as a minimum GPA.

Post-Professional Programs

Some physical therapists want advanced training to build their skills after graduation. This type of education is termed "post-professional." The first kind of post-professional training is a clinical residency program. Most residencies last about one year and are designed to provide additional training and experience in specialty areas of practice. After completing a residency program, PTs can choose to go even further and pursue a fellowship program. Fellowships provide intensive instruction within a subspecialty area of practice. They usually include extensive mentored clinical experience.

Licenses and Certifications

Physical therapists in all 50 states must be licensed in order to practice. Licensing requirements vary by state, but all include passing the National Physical Therapy Examination. The exam is conducted by the Federation of State Boards of Physical Therapy (FSBPT). A law exam and a criminal background check are required by some states. Continuing education is necessary for physical therapists to keep their license in most states.

After gaining work experience, many physical therapists choose to become specialists. It is not necessary to be certified in order to practice in a specific area. There are many types of physical therapy and certification is only offered for nine of them. Even for those nine, certification is voluntary. Most PTs practicing in a specialty, however, have obtained advanced training, such as one of these accredited residency programs.

Specialty certification is currently offered in the following areas:

- Cardiovascular and Pulmonary
- Clinical Electrophysiology
- Geriatrics
- Neurology
- Orthopaedics
- Pediatrics
- Sports Physical Therapy
- Women's Health
- The ninth area, oncology, is scheduled for 2019.

To become a board-certified specialist, PTs must pass an exam administered by the American Board of Physical Therapy Specialties. Individuals are eligible to take the exam after completing 2,000 hours of clinical work or by completing a residency program accredited by the American Physical Therapy Association (APTA). Either experience must be focused in the specialty area.

EARNINGS

THE DEMAND FOR QUALIFIED PHYSICAL THERAPISTS has continually pushed salaries for these professionals upwards in recent years, and the trend is not likely to stop anytime soon. Currently, the median annual income of physical therapists is about $85,000, with the most common salary range on a national level being $75,000 to $100,000. Only the lowest 10 percent earn less than $60,000. Actual income depends on a variety of factors, including work setting, geographic area, and experience. With the right combination, top salaries can reach $120,000.

Most physical therapists work in one of five settings. Here are the median annual salaries in those settings:

- Home healthcare services
  $90,000

- $83,000

- Physical, occupational, and speech therapy clinics
  $ 80,000

- Nursing care facilities
  $90,000

- General hospitals
  $85,000

- Private medical offices
  $83,000

- Physical, occupational, and speech therapy clinics

  $80,000

Salaries can vary greatly from one area to the next. For example, the average PT salary in Montana is $70,000, but the average in Nevada is almost $125,000. Salaries also vary within states, even from town to town. If you intend to move to a new location after you graduate, it would be wise to carefully research possible destinations. One way to check out new locations is to sign up with a traveling PT agency. Traveling PTs have the advantage of earning top dollar no matter where their contracts take them. The average salary of around $100,000 is significantly higher compared to permanent positions. Plus, these jobs often provide additional benefits, such as transportation, food, and housing.

Experience matters, but even new PTs do well. Entry-level jobs for physical therapists with fewer than three years of experience pay $60,000 on average. The overall median salary of $85,000 can be attained within a few years, and the salaries continue to go up the longer someone is in the profession.

Most physical therapists work full time, regardless of whether they are salaried or paid by the hour. Only one in five works part time. Full-time workers usually receive benefits, such as health insurance, sick leave, and retirement plans from their employers. Those working part time may not receive full benefits.

OPPORTUNITIES

THE EMPLOYMENT OUTLOOK FOR PHYSICAL THERAPISTS is exceptionally good. The number of jobs is expected to grow more than 35 percent over the coming decade. That is much faster than the average for all occupations. In fact, it is among the 20 fastest-growing careers. The job outlook for aides and assistants is even better – about 40 percent. Demand is high and unemployment low across the board, but that does vary by geographic location and type of practice.

The sunny outlook for job prospects is further bolstered by a growing shortage of qualified applicants. The APTA has pointed out that even though the number of physical therapy students has been on the rise, the demand will continue to outpace the number of trained physical therapists entering the workforce well into the future.

Job opportunities are expected to be good for licensed physical therapists in all settings. However, projected job growth is better in certain healthcare sectors. A great number of physical therapists currently work at hospitals or are self-employed, yet those two healthcare segments are expected to add fewer new jobs compared to home healthcare services, offices of physicians, and nursing care facilities. The most job growth for physical therapists is projected to be in therapy offices that provide physical, occupational, and/or speech therapy.

One major reason for the growing demand for physical therapists is the aging of the US population. The baby boomer generation, which includes about 75 million people, started turning 65 in 2011. Since then, *10,000 more have turned 65 every day*. Older people, in general, are more likely to experience strokes, heart attacks, and mobility-related injuries that require physical therapy for recovery. Baby boomers are also staying more active later in life than their counterparts of previous generations. Their aging bodies are more likely to succumb to sports related injuries. Overall, there should be particularly good job prospects wherever the elderly are likely to be treated, such as acute care hospitals, skilled nursing facilities, and orthopedic practices.

The incidence of chronic conditions, such as diabetes, rheumatoid arthritis, and obesity has been rapidly increasing in recent years. There are almost 30 million people in the US with diabetes. For these people, physical therapists and PTAs can be life-changers. More physical therapists are needed to help them maintain their mobility and manage the effects of their chronic conditions.

Physical therapists will continue to help patients recover more quickly from surgery. Advances in medical technology have led to an increased use of outpatient surgery to treat injuries and illnesses. Short-term physical therapy often follows outpatient surgery to obtain the best results and to avoid the need for hospitalization.

Due to medical and technological developments, a greater percentage of people born with permanent disabilities and babies born with birth defects are able to survive. Likewise, in cases of traumatic injuries that might have resulted in death in the past, there is a much better chance of recovery today. There is an increasing need for physical therapists who can help enable individuals with long-term conditions to function better in their daily lives.

Greater access to health insurance has also contributed to the demand for physical therapy services. Due to federal health insurance reform, more than 20 million people who were previously uninsured are now covered. That means these individuals, who might not have been able to get therapeutic treatments before, can now obtain the assistance of physical therapists.

Job prospects for physical therapists have always varied by geographic location. That will not change. Generally, though, prospects are more favorable in rural areas since so many physical therapists are competing for positions in highly populated cities and suburban areas.

GETTING STARTED

YOU HAVE WORKED HARD TO GET THROUGH COLLEGE and now you are ready to kick start your new career. If you were smart, you started laying the foundation for your career long before graduation. Employers like to see experience, even from newly licensed PTs. One of the best ways to get that experience is through an internship. This is often unpaid work, but that does not matter. It looks great on a résumé – in fact, employers expect to see at least one internship. More than one is even better. There are many internship programs available through hospitals, rehabilitation centers, nursing homes, and clinics. The easiest way to find them is to enlist the help of your college counselor.

As you start your search, you can rest assured that jobs will definitely be available. Prospects are expected to be good for licensed physical therapists in all settings, however, actual job growth will be much greater in some healthcare industry segments than in others. Job seekers who are knowledgeable about where the highest growth is taking place will definitely be at an advantage. Look at offices providing physical, occupational and/or speech therapy, where you will find the greatest number of opportunities. Job openings will also be plentiful in home healthcare services, and nursing care facilities and other places where the elderly are being cared for.

Before researching job ads online and in newspapers, do some research into these fast-growing segments. You are likely to uncover job opportunities that have not yet been announced to the public. Instead of waiting for a job opening to be advertised or posted online, go straight to the source. Apply directly to clinics, private practices, and healthcare facilities that have the most need of more physical therapists. Target these prospective employers directly with a résumé tailored to fit their particular type of practice. You can easily do this online through sites like LinkedIn.

Continue your job search online and offline. Your school's job placement center will have listings. So will the state employment office and the classified section of your local paper. There are employment agencies, both on the Internet and off, that specialize in health related jobs. There are also industry associations, such as APTA, devoted to the physical therapy profession, that post jobs from all over the country.

While looking for your first job, maintain a regular exercise routine. You will want to be in excellent shape once hired so you can keep up with the physical rigors of the job.

ASSOCIATIONS

■ **American Physical Therapy Association**
http://www.apta.org

■ **Commission on Accreditation in Physical Therapy Education**
http://www.capteonline.org

■ **American Board of Physical Therapy Specialties**
http://www.abpts.org

■ **Physical Therapist Centralized Application Service (PTCAS)**
www.ptcas.org

■ **Federation of State Boards of Physical Therapy**
https://www.fsbpt.org/

PERIODICALS

■ **Physical Therapy Journal**
http://ptjournal.apta.org

■ **Journal of Orthopaedic & Sports Physical Therapy**
http://www.jospt.org/

WEBSITES

■ **Physical Therapy Assistant Jobs**
http://physical-therapy-assistant.org/pta-jobs

■ **PT Jobs**
http://www.ptjobs.com

■ **Physical Therapist**
https://www.physicaltherapist.com/physical-therapy-jobs

■ **Physical Therapy Now**
http://www.ptnow.org

Copyright 2017
Institute For Career Research

CAREERS REPORTS
www.amazon.com/author/careers

CAREERS INTERNET DATABASE
www.careers-internet.org

Information
service@careers-internet.org

www.ingramcontent.com/pod-product-compliance
Lightning Source LLC
Chambersburg PA
CBHW061237180526

45170CB00003B/1336